FREE
DVD

DVD

From Stress to Success DVD from Trivium Test Prep

Dear Customer,

Thank you for purchasing from Trivium Test Prep! Whether you're looking to join the military, get into college, or advance your career, we're honored to be a part of your journey.

To show our appreciation (and to help you relieve a little of that test-prep stress), we're offering a **FREE *ACSM Essential Test Tips DVD*** by Trivium Test Prep. Our DVD includes 35 test preparation strategies that will help keep you calm and collected before and during your big exam. All we ask is that you email us your feedback and describe your experience with our product. Amazing, awful, or just so-so: we want to hear what you have to say!

To receive your **FREE *ACSM Essential Test Tips DVD***, please email us at 5star@triviumtestprep.com. Include "Free 5 Star" in the subject line and the following information in your email:

1. The title of the product you purchased.
2. Your rating from 1 – 5 (with 5 being the best).
3. Your feedback about the product, including how our materials helped you meet your goals and ways in which we can improve our products.
4. Your full name and shipping address so we can send your **FREE *ACSM Essential Test Tips DVD***.

If you have any questions or concerns please feel free to contact us directly at 5star@triviumtestprep.com. Thank you, and good luck with your studies!

* Please note that the free DVD is <u>not included</u> with this book. To receive the free DVD, please follow the instructions above.

ACSM CERTIFICATION REVIEW BOOK OF FLASH CARDS

ACSM Test Prep Review with 300+ Flash Cards for the American College of Sports Medicine Certified Personal Trainer Exam

TABLE OF CONTENTS

INTRODUCTION

What is a Personal Trainer?

The world of personal training is vast and growing in many ways. A personal trainer is an educated exercise professional who possesses the knowledge and skill set to create and instruct others in various fitness-related settings. Personal trainers must strive to achieve a base of knowledge and to acquire the skills to properly design and implement research-based training programs that are safe and effective for their clientele. It is up to the certified personal trainer to ensure the client receives the highest quality training experience through appropriate goal setting, needs analysis, exercise prescriptions, and health and fitness education. Additionally, it is the certified personal trainer's responsibility to develop and employ these methods within his or her scope of practice. There are a variety of different career paths a certified personal trainer can pursue based on his or her interests and abilities.

Personal trainers can be productive in many different settings and businesses. The most common settings in which personal trainers work are the large, well-known gym chains and smaller, privately owned fitness centers that are common in the United States. These facilities are generally open to hiring newly trained, certified fitness professionals and are a good starting point for anyone looking to advance within a specific company.

However, there are a number of other settings in which certified personal trainers can utilize their health and fitness knowledge. For example, personal trainers can work in clinical settings, corporate training, in-home private settings, sports camps, and more. Working in a clinical setting as a personal trainer often involves administering exercise stress tests with a team supervised by a physician or medical practitioner. Corporate trainers tend to work at the private fitness centers of corporations in an office building. Some clientele prefer a more personalized workout within the privacy of their own home; the certified personal trainer will travel to the client's house with his or her equipment. Depending on the fitness professional's background, it may be preferable to work as a sports-specific strength and conditioning coach. There are many career paths available, but one key component of the personal training world is the certification.

American College of Sports Medicine (ACSM)

The **American College of Sports Medicine (ACSM)** is another of the oldest professional fitness organizations in the field of exercise science and is recognized as a gold standard in health and fitness. Developed in the 1950s, the ACSM is a worldwide association of over 50,000 members. The organization was developed by physicians and fitness professionals working together to provide the highest-quality research in the field of sports medicine and exercise. The ACSM offers a variety of certifications for all levels of education and various specializations and credential programs. ACSM certifications include certified personal trainer (CPT), certified group exercise instructor (GEI), and certified exercise physiologist (EP-C). ACSM advanced certifications include certified clinical exercise physiologist (CEP) requiring a bachelor's degree in exercise science and clinical work experience, as well as registered certified exercise physiologist (RCEP) requiring a graduate degree and experience overseeing clinical exercise testing. Like the NSCA, the ACSM has been devoted to producing science-based research journals in sports medicine and exercise science for decades and is seen as one of the leaders in fitness education worldwide. The main goal of the ACSM is to develop the most scientifically relevant research, methods, and application of their research to the entirety of the health and fitness industry.

ACSM Test Details

The ACSM tests are broken up into different domains testing various exercise-science–related aspects. The Certified Personal Trainer (ACSM—CPT) exam has 150 questions split into four testing domains: Initial Client Consultation and Assessment; Exercise Program Design and Implementation; Exercise Leadership and Client Education; and Legal, Professional, Business, and Marketing. Candidates have two hours and thirty minutes to complete the ACSM—CPT exam and receive test results immediately.

What's on the ACSM Certification Exams?

Domain	Number of Questions	Percentage
Initial Client Consultation and Assessment	39	26%
Exercise Program Design and Implementation	41 (approx.)	27%
Exercise Leadership and Client Education	40 (approx.)	27%
Legal, Professional, Business, and Marketing	30	20%
Total:	150 questions	2 hours and 30 minutes

Questions in Domain I, Initial Client Consultation and Assessment, require you to show your ability to gather health and exercise history information, use interviews and questionnaires, and assess clients' current physical capabilities, attitudes, and goals for effective program design. For Domain II, Exercise Program Design and Implementation, examinees must be able to interpret the results of assessments to design exercise programs for clients based on their goals. Review the FITTE principle to prepare for this section of the test. Questions may ask about training methods, periodization, biomechanics, establishing and monitoring exercise intensity, program design for special populations, modifications, and other issues. You may also encounter questions about safe training and spotting practices, and signs of contraindications. For Exercise Leadership and Client Education, Domain III, prepare to demonstrate your knowledge about communication, motivation, and client education. Finally, Domain IV, Legal, Professional, Business, and Marketing, covers topics including the use of ACSM guidelines to obtain medical clearance for exercise programs, risk management, scope of practice, working with healthcare professionals, the ACSM Code of Ethics, and business issues, among others.

Each multiple-choice question is worth one raw point. The total number of questions you answer correctly is added up to obtain your raw score, which is then converted to a scale of 200 – 800. A passing score is 550 or higher. Scores are broken down by content area on score reports, so candidates can determine strengths and weaknesses. To register for an ACSM certification exam, visit the certification section on the ACSM website. This redirects to a separate page with additional information regarding the ACSM examination process and registration. The examination is taken either at a third-party certified testing center or at university testing centers. You will require a valid photo ID. ACSM members receive a discounted exam fee.

ONE: FLASH CARDS

What is the biological hierarchy?

Ligaments are tissues that
attach bones to what?

The biological hierarchy is a systematic breakdown of the structures of the human body and is typically organized from smallest to largest or largest to smallest (i.e., cells to organism or organism to cells).

other bones

What are examples of hinge joints?

In which anatomical direction does scoliosis occur at the spine?

What major effect does axial loading have on the human skeletal system?

elbows, knees, and most fingers (excluding the thumbs)

lateral

improving bone mineral density to delay the onset of osteoporosis

The I-band of a sarcomere
contains which filaments?

What is the purpose of muscle
spindle fibers?

Due to their mode of sustained duration
training, ultra-marathon athletes
will primarily have an abundance
of which type of muscle fibers?

actin filaments

Muscle spindle fibers are proprioceptors that sense a stretch in the muscle. They create a subsequent neuromotor response that causes the muscular contraction of the agonist muscle and reciprocal inhibition of the antagonist muscle.

type I, slow-twitch muscle fibers

Do type II, fast-twitch muscle fibers have a higher or lower density of mitochondria than type I, slow-twitch muscle fibers?

What is the difference between muscular hypertrophy and muscular hyperplasia?

Does the pulmonary artery carry oxygenated or deoxygenated blood to the lungs?

Type II, fast-twitch muscle fibers have a *lower* density of mito-chondria than type I, slow-twitch muscle fibers.

Muscular hypertrophy refers to an increase in the *size* of the muscle fibers; muscular hyperplasia refers to an increase in the *number* of muscle fibers.

deoxygenated blood

What is the most common type of COPD that fitness professionals will encounter? (It is typically exacerbated by exercise.)

Which type of lever system does a calf raise (standing on the balls of the feet) use?

When the body is producing ATP via creatine phosphate and/or muscle glycogen stores, which energy system is being utilized?

asthma

A calf raise uses the second-class lever system: the calf muscles are the muscular force; the resistive force is the weight of the body; and the fulcrum is the ball of the foot (force, resistance, fulcrum).

the anaerobic energy system

To meet the needs of the exercising muscle, anaerobic glycolysis produces excessive amounts of hydrogen ions in the bloodstream due to lack of oxygen uptake. What is the byproduct?

What is EPOC?

Which part of the nervous system is responsible for the "fight-or-flight" response?

lactic acid

EPOC is *excessive post-exercise oxygen consumption*, and it is the body's continued consumption of oxygen following exercise resulting in more energy expenditure, even at rest.

somatic nervous system

Which part of the nervous system is responsible for the "rest and digest" response?

Which plane of motion and muscular actions occur as a result of the contraction of the quadriceps muscles?

Why should equipment and floors at the training facility be cleaned regularly?

autonomic nervous system

plane of motion: sagittal; muscular action: hip flexion and/or knee extension

Cleaning prevents the spread of infectious disease and bacteria.

In a third-class lever system, where is the muscular force located in relation to the fulcrum and resistance?

Which hormone is responsible for the regulation of heart rate, blood pressure, and more due to autonomic responses to stimuli?

How does exercise benefit the cardiovascular system?

The muscular force is located in the middle of the fulcrum and resistance.

epinephrine

Exercise improves heart efficiency and capillary density; it also decreases blood pressure and increases blood volume.

Vitamins are divided into
which two categories?

Are vitamins and minerals considered
macronutrients or micronutrients?

Which macronutrient is the body's
primary source for sustained, long-
duration, low-intensity exercise?

water soluble and fat soluble

micronutrients

fats

How many kcals does each
macronutrient provide per
gram of nutrient?

What are the main electrolytes
lost through sweat?

How many grams of protein per
kilogram of body weight are
recommended for endurance-
based athletes? What about
strength-based athletes?

carbohydrates: 4 kcals/gram
fats: 9 kcals/gram
proteins: 4 kcals/gram

---

sodium and potassium

1.2 – 1.4 g/kg for endurance-based athletes; 1.6 – 1.7 g/kg
for strength-based athletes

Which type of athlete benefits most from a carbohydrate-loading dietary routine?

Which eating disorder is characterized by an overwhelming urge to binge followed by compensatory purging through fasting, excessive exercise, use of laxatives, or vomiting?

According to normative standards, what is the range of BMI that is considered overweight?

Endurance athletes benefit from carbohydrate-loading.

bulimia nervosa

25.0 – 29.9

Why do fitness professionals perform an exercise assessment with clients?

How does pre-testing prior to the start of a fitness program help the fitness professional?

When should flexibility training be completed during a workout?

An exercise assessment helps determine a client's past and present health as well as their current fitness level. Exercise assessments also help the client set realistic and achievable goals.

Pre-testing helps the fitness professional determine the client's basic abilities and design an exercise program that accommodates their training level and goals.

at the end of a workout; muscles become more elastic after exercise

Why should a fitness professional use a medical history form to determine which medications, if any, a client is taking?

What does a static postural assessment help the fitness professional determine?

What are the three components assessed by overhead squat assessment tests?

Some medications can affect physiological factors, such as resting heart rate, exercising heart rate, and blood pressure.

This assessment reveals whether the client has any muscular imbalances, joint misalignments, or tight musculature that may impact their ability to perform certain exercises.

neuromuscular efficiency, functional strength, and dynamic flexibility

What does the bilateral
broad jump assess?

Which athletes benefit from having
their vertical jump height assessed?

Which type of athletic ability does
the pro-agility test measure?

total body bilateral power

athletes participating in sports that require lower body power and vertical jumping movements, such as basketball, volleyball, or high-jump

lateral speed and agility

What test measures the static flexibility of the low back and hamstrings muscle groups?

Which anatomical sites are used when measuring the resting heart rate?

Which measurement in mmHg indicates healthy blood pressure?

the sit-and-reach test

the neck or the wrist, to measure the carotid pulse or radial pulse, respectively

~120/80 mmHg

What do the air displacement plethysmography, bioelectrical impedance analysis, and dual-energy X-ray absorptiometry assessments measure?

What three sites are typically used for skinfold measurements when assessing body fat percentage with skinfold calipers in men? In women?

Which assessment is used to determine a client's maximal strength in a particular exercise, and how is this test beneficial?

body composition

---

men: quadriceps, abdominal, pectoral
women: quadriceps, above the hip, triceps

The one-repetition maximum test (1RM) can help determine the client's maximal strength in a particular movement as well as calculate weight at various repetition ranges. It can also be used as an assessment tool to see improvements in muscular strength.

What remains constant in an isokinetic muscular contraction?

Which muscles act as synergists and primary movers in the squat exercise?

What is the primary goal of warming up prior to starting a workout?

the rate of force application

---

hamstrings and quadriceps

Warming up increases the range of motion of the muscles, allowing proper neuromuscular efficiency.

What is the purpose of performing self-myofascial release (SMR) techniques at the start of a workout?

Which dynamic stretching exercise might be used to increase activation of the glutes, hamstrings, hip flexors, and quadriceps muscles?

Which muscle groups does the straight-leg march, a dynamic stretch, attempt to activate?

SMR techniques help initiate autogenic inhibition of the Golgi tendon organs, releasing tension in the muscle and increasing range of motion.

lunge walks or walking knee lifts

the hip flexors, core, and hamstring muscles

Which muscle groups are primarily targeted by the lateral pulldown exercise?

The back-loaded squat exercise primarily targets which muscle groups?

How would an individual act as a spotter for the back-loaded barbell squat exercise?

the latissimus dorsi and posterior deltoids

the glutes, hamstrings, quadriceps, and erector spinae

The spotter should be positioned behind the exerciser. The spotter should mimic the squat movement with arms positioned under the armpits of the exerciser to guide and maintain torso integrity, protecting the exerciser's lower back.

Resisted or assisted sprinting drills are examples of what type of training?

What do plyometric training drills primarily focus on?

Would the cone drill, also known as the T-drill, have a greater benefit for a triathlete or a soccer player? Why?

overspeed training

Plyometric training drills primarily focus on explosive movement or maximal force production in the least amount of time.

Cone drills benefit soccer players more than triathletes because soccer requires a significant amount of lateral movement, speed, and agility.

Which piece of cardiovascular equipment is considered more advanced: the stair climber or the recumbent bicycle?

Which form of cardiovascular exercise has the least impact on the joints and is most beneficial to those with joint issues in the lower extremities: walking, jogging, sprinting, or swimming?

What are the primary muscle groups targeted in the leg press exercise?

the stair climber

swimming

glutes, hamstrings, and quadriceps muscles

When designing a training program, what does the *training stimulus* refer to?

Why is it necessary to provide a full day of recovery before performing resistance training exercises on the same muscle groups?

When should the trainer look to increase the intensity of a specific exercise?

the types of exercises applied in the program

A day of recovery is necessary to avoid overtraining or overuse injuries, which can limit progress.

when the client has reached a high level of proficiency with the current exercise

Where are measurements
for the waist taken?

What is the proper regression of a
back-loaded barbell squat exercise?

Which declines more rapidly due to
the effect of detraining: muscular
fitness or cardiovascular fitness?

at the narroest point of the waist or, when there is no narrowing, directly around the navel

body weight squats, wall sits, or dumbbell squats (suitcase squat)

Cardiovascular fitness declines more rapidly; muscular fitness declines gradually.

What is a progression of the standard push-up exercise?

How does vertical loading differ from horizontal loading?

Microcycles are typically associated with phases of training programs aimed at specific adaptations; what are the different types of phases?

plyometric push-ups, archer push-ups, elevated leg push-ups

Vertical loading minimizes rest periods by selecting varying muscle groups through a circuit of exercises, allowing one muscle group a chance to rest while another is functioning. Horizontal loading exercises a muscle group consecutively and requires rest periods between the sets.

---

endurance phase, hypertrophy phase, strength phase, and power phase

What should a transition phase
in the off-season incorporate?

Why is resistance training for muscular
endurance NOT recommended for an
athlete during the competitive season?

How many sets and repetitions should
clients seeking to improve muscular
strength incorporate in resistance
training exercises? How long should
their rest period be? At what load
should these exercises be done?

an active rest period with no resistance training or high-performance competition

Resistance training contributes to excessive fatigue that can hinder the athlete's performance in competition.

three to five sets with one to eight repetitions
Up to three minutes of rest
80 – 100 percent of 1RM

Which guideline of sets, repetitions, rest period, and load should clients seeking to improve muscular endurance follow?

Which exercises might help clients achieve muscular balance if their program already incorporates significant use of the chest, triceps, and anterior deltoid muscles?

Based on the principle of specificity, would an ice hockey player benefit more from the bench press exercise or the barbell back squat exercise? Why?

one to three sets, fifteen or more repetitions, with thirty or fewer seconds of rest at 60 – 70% of 1RM

---

exercises that focus on the back, biceps, and posterior deltoids, such as bent-over rows, seated rows, lateral pulldowns, or the rear fly exercise

---

The barbell back squat exercise would offer a greater benefit because it uses the primary muscle groups associated with skating and partially mimics the squatted stance associated with skating. The bench press supports the back and places emphasis on the chest and triceps, which are not as significantly important in the movements of the sport.

Why is it important to perform exercises from *higher* intensity to *lower* intensity (following a dynamic warm-up) rather than from *lower* intensity to *higher* intensity?

What should an cardiovascular training program for children primarily focus on?

What should strength training programs for children emphasize?

Higher-intensity exercises require a significant amount of technique and energy from the muscles. If the lower-intensity exercises are performed first, fatigue may impact the client's ability to perform the exercise properly, increasing risk of injury.

developing technique and coordination; preventing long-term overuse

form and technique

Which type of exercise should
be prohibited when training
a pregnant woman?

Which exercises should
obese clients avoid?

How can the fitness professional
modify cardiovascular activities
for individuals with COPD?

Any type of exercise that could put the fetus at risk of injury, such as non-stationary cycling and contact sports, should be avoided.

An obese client should avoid high-impact exercises and exercise in the heat to prevent strain on the joints, overheating, and difficulty breathing.

by reducing the time per session of cardiovascular exercise

On average, at least how often should resistance training be performed?

On average, at least how often should cardiovascular training be performed?

Posture, gestures, facial expressions, eye movements, and tone of voice are all examples of what type of communication?

two to three times per week

three to five days a week

body language—nonverbal communication

Clients in the cognitive stage of learning will benefit most from which types of exercise?

What type of feedback relates to improvements in kinesthetic awareness to correct motor function?

What is the typical work-to-rest ratio for clients who are just starting an exercise program?

simple, basic exercises with light weights and simple movement patterns to help build neuromuscular efficiency and kinesthetic awareness

internal feedback

1:1

What are the stages of the
readiness-to-change theory?

During which stage of change
does the client begin to initiate a
connection by asking questions
to identify areas of concern?

During which stage of change do clients
reach their goals and become ready to
independently enjoy a healthy lifestyle?

precontemplation, contemplation, preparation, action, maintenance, termination

preparation

termination

Which additional certifications may benefit the fitness professional in the event of an emergency?

Why is it important for a fitness professional to understand the various forms of negligence in the fitness center?

Name several components of an appropriate emergency action plan.

CPR, AED, and first aid training

Negligence is a common reason for lawsuits and can occur in numerous aspects of the fitness field.

---

a method of signaling emergency services

a procedure outlining an evacuation or emergency escape route

assigning tasks to employees to ensure conditions do not become more hazardous for emergency responders

a method to ensure all employees are evacuated safely

direct resources for first responders

a list of employees and their designated responsibilities during an emergency

Clients who suffer from generalized fatigue, poor sleep, depression, chronic muscle soreness and joint pain, decreases in physical performance, or an increase in resting heart rate, but who still train regularly, are exhibiting what?

Overtraining is often a result of what?

What is the peak timeframe for the onset of DOMS?

overtraining

lacking adequate rest or recovery between workout sessions

twenty-four to forty-eight hours after a workout

When should a client see a doctor about a musculoskeletal injury?

What does the fitness professional's scope of practice include?

What is muscular hypertrophy?

A client should see a doctor if the client's pain, swelling, or other symptoms persist for longer than a few days, if movement produces grating, popping, or crackling sounds, or if there are unusual sensations under the skin.

exercise program design, fitness assessments, exercise technique, body composition measurement, fitness goal setting, exercise adherence, and motivational methods

an increase in the size of muscle cells

Which assessment is used to determine upper body strength?

What muscular action occurs as a limb is pulled toward the midline of the body?

An Olympic weightlifter who attempts a single repetition of an exercise for competition would benefit most from having which type of muscle?

The bench press test is used to determine upper body strength.

adduction

type IIb muscle fibers (for maximal power output)

Muscular atrophy occurs
as a result of what?

What is the difference between a
macromineral and a micromineral?

During a gait assessment, the personal
trainer should use the lateral view to
check which kinetic chain checkpoint?

injury or lack of exercise

Macrominerals are typically present in the body in larger quantities than microminerals and have larger dietary requirements.

head, low back, and shoulders

Which joint allows for the most freedom of movement?

How much time should an American adult commit to exercise each week?

What is the single-leg squat test used to assess?

Ball-and-socket joints allow for the most freedom of movement.

A weekly total of 2.5 hours is the standard amount of exercise recommended for American adults.

single-leg strength

To ensure accurate results, the resting heart rate should be taken at what time of the day?

What is the term that describes the reason for an individual's action?

What happens to a person's base of support when their feet are spread farther apart?

upon rising in the morning, for three consecutive days

motivation

The base of support increases with a wider foot stance.

When taking a circumference measurement of the thigh, where should the tape measure be positioned?

Which questionnaire identifies injury or previous surgery?

During exercise that lasts over one hour, how much fluid intake is recommended to maintain hydration?

10 inches above the patella

a medical history questionnaire

20 – 36 oz. of fluid, preferably a sport drink with electrolytes, at intervals of fifteen to twenty minutes——

What is the strongest predictor of
exercise program adherence?

What is multiple sclerosis?

What is the glycemic index?

exercise history—it will detail previous exercise habits

Multiple sclerosis is a disease that affects the myelin sheaths on axons.

The glycemic index is the area under the blood glucose curve (AUC) over a two-hour time period following ingestion of the food, divided by the AUC of a standard food (usually white bread) times 100.

Why is it important to consider client enjoyment when designing an exercise program?

What is the proper rest period between sets of deadlifts at five repetitions and heavy loads?

How can a trainer tell if the client is legitimately at an eight or nine on the RPE scale?

Clients who enjoy exercise are more likely to be compliant.

At heavy loads and low volumes, rest periods should be three minutes.

The client will not be able to complete sentences because the intensity will be so high.

What is typical of an athlete's training program during the preperatory period?

What type of training uses controlled instability to increase proprioception?

Which postural misalignment is characterized by rounded shoulders and a forward head position?

Training is at a lower intensity, focuses on building strength, and may not be sport specific.

core training

upper crossed syndrome

What does proper breathing
technique control?

During the three-minute step test,
the metronome should be set to
how many beats per minute?

A foam roller is used for
what type of training?

Proper breathing technique controls core activation, repetition tempo, and range of motion.

ninety-six beats per minute

self-myofascial release

Advanced lifters who are lifting heavy loads adopt which type of breathing technique?

What do tendons connect?

Which test is most suitable to assess lower body strength: the barbell squat or the overhead squat?

the Valsalva breathing maneuver

Ligaments connect muscles to bones.

The barbell squat test is used to measure lower body strength. The overhead squat test assesses dynamic flexibility.

In a standing or sitting position, a client should maintain which three points of contact?

What are open kinetic chain exercises?

What is characteristic of workouts during an athlete's competitive period?

The client's head, shoulders, and glutes should maintain contact with the wall or dowel.

exercises that allow foot or hand movement

The competitive period is the athlete's peak season; workouts typically focus on sport-specific training and/or maintenance of fitness at moderate intensity.

If the rest period is around thirty seconds and the load is light, which repetition range is most appropriate?

An effective warm-up should last between five and ten minutes at what type of intensity?

When spotting a shoulder press, where should the spotter's hands be?

For short rest periods and light loads, fifteen repetitions are appropriate.

low to moderate intensity

The spotter should support the elbows.

What types of exercises are considered dynamic stretches?

The sit-and-reach test measures the flexibility of what muscles?

What must a trainer require from any client who discloses potentially serious health conditions during an initial meeting to discuss a fitness program?

butt kickers, prisoner squats (lower limbs); arm circles, medicine ball chop/lifts (upper limbs)

lower back and hamstring

Physician clearance should be required prior to beginning an exercise program for safety reasons.

What is the primary training emphasis
in the power phase of fitness training?

Which is an alternative to
standard aerobic training?

Which behavior change model focuses on
understanding the relationship between
a person and his or her environment?

muscle speed and force production

circuit training, which can use various exercises in a continuous sequence with minimal rest, causing an elevated heart rate for an extended period

the socio-ecological model

What is a regression of a
kettlebell swing?

What is the primary mover
for a wrist curl?

What is a regression for a push press?

a straight leg deadlift

the forearm

a seated dumbbell shoulder press

What are the three top accredited certifying agencies that set the standards of practice for the fitness industry?

Inconsistency of a muscle around a joint is considered a

_____.

A floor crunch is a regression for what core exercise?

NASM, ACE, and ACSM are the three top agencies in personal training certification.

muscle imbalance

ball crunch

What grip is used primarily in parallel bar or dumbbell pushing and pulling movements, where the thumbs stay up and the palms face each other?

When is the first transition period of an athlete's exercise program?

What should an effective cooldown do?

neutral grip

just before the start of the season or competition

An effective cooldown mimics the warm-up to ensure a steady reduction in heart rate.

What is a regression for a ball crunch?

Football players run one hundred yards at most. Following the principle of specificity, should the trainer implement long-distance running in the training program?

Performing a specific number of repetitions through the full range of motion is called what?

abdominal crunch

No. Long-distance running does not follow the principle of specificity when it comes to football.

a set

What is the range of movement
for hinge joints?

When should a personal trainer
prematurely terminate a
cardiorespiratory assessment?

What should resistance training
programs for children and
adolescents focus on?

flexion and extension

in case of emergency or when the client asks to stop

proper technique and form

Is a pronated grip underhanded or overhanded?

A muscular contraction in which the rate of force application remains constant is called what?

What test is the most important indicator of a client's ability to complete the activities of daily living?

overhanded

isokinetic

the cardiorespiratory test, which assesses an individual's maximal oxygen consumption

If a client had a recent joint surgery, what should he or she do before starting a fitness program?

When should PNF stretching be implemented into the program?

How do novice clients' rest periods differ from those of advanced clients?

The client should obtain a physician's clearance to participate in an exercise program that incorporates that joint.

PNF stretching should be saved for the end of the workout to improve flexibility.

Because novice clients lack conditioning, they may require more frequent and longer rest periods than advanced clients do.

Along with proper body positioning, another way to isolate muscle groups with efficiency is to use different types of _____ while lifting barbells, dumbbells, or kettlebells, and while using weight machines.

A muscular contraction that is being performed at the same force throughout range of motion is called what?

What does the 1RM test measure?

grips

isotonic

The 1RM test measures the client's ability to perform an exercise at the maximal effort of strength for a single repetition.

What happens to heart rate and respiration rate during both aerobic and anaerobic exercise?

What does CEC stand for?

What is the second transition period?

Both heart rate and respiration rate should increase during aerobic and anaerobic cardiovascular exercise.

CEC stands for *continuing education credit.*

The second transition period is a time of active recovery that includes recreational activities not related to the athlete's competition.

In a training program, what does a superset refer to?

What is self-efficacy?

A muscular contraction in which the resistance and force are even and no movement is taking place is called what?

performing an exercise and then immediately performing another exercise utilizing the antagonist, or opposite muscle groups

Self-efficacy is the ability to believe in oneself to achieve a goal.

isometric

Injury is a _____ factor that can be a barrier to exercise adherence.

A muscular contraction in which the muscle resists a force as it lengthens is called what?

What is the repetition range for development of muscular hypertrophy?

physical-activity

eccentric

eight to twelve repetitions

The client masters an exercise technique without movement compensations. What learning stage is the client in?

Which test is used to measure maximal speed?

How should the trainer modify abdominal exercises, such as the crunch, for pregnant clients?

the autonomous stage of learning

the forty-yard dash

The trainer should seat the pregnant client slightly upright for abdominal exercises.

Income is categorized as which type of barrier to exercise adherence?

Does detraining occur more quickly in resistance training gains or cardiovascular training gains?

What should be done in addition to dynamic stretching during the warm-up process?

Income is a personal attribute that can be a barrier to exercise adherence.

cardiovascular training gains, which may suffer substantial losses just two weeks after training cessation

light to moderate cardiovascular exercise

A muscular contraction in which the length of the muscle shortens to lift the resistance is called what?

One major advantage of zone training in cardiovascular exercise programs is that

What kinds of exercises should program design for senior citizens incorporate?

concentric

It provides exercise variance through different target heart rate zones and keeps the program interesting for the client.

Exercises that make the activities of daily living easier should be incorporated into programs for senior citizens, especially exercises that help prevent injuries and falls.

People who believe that their lives are controlled by what happens to them have an _____ locus of control.

How many American adults get the minimum recommended levels of activity, according to the CDC?

What can the trainer implement to improve the client's lactate threshold?

external

45 percent

sprint interval training

According to the CDC, what percentage
of adults in the US are obese?

Where should the rules and
regulations for an emergency
action plan be obtained?

Fifty percent of individuals adhering
to a fitness program drop out
after what period of time?

34 percent

the US Department of Labor

six months

In the _____ phase of change, the individual has taken definitive steps to change his or her behavior.

Because of an increased Q-angle, female athletes are at a higher risk of medial knee injuries in which sport(s)?

A trainer who provides advice or information beyond their certified or licensed specialty is working outside of their _____.

action phase

basketball, volleyball, and any other sports involving jumping

scope of practice

What is the term for positive feedback emphasizing a specific aspect of an individual's behavior or action?

Miscellaneous personal trainer's insurance covers which type of claim?

When an individual initiates a plan to solve a problem within a month, that person is in the _____ phase.

targeted praise

bodily injury

preparation

What does READ stand for?

What impact can anabolic steroid abuse have on the liver?

The RICE method of treatment is appropriate for what types of injuries?

Rapport, Empathy, Assessment, Development

Anabolic steroid abuse can damage the liver.

sprains, strains, or contusions

What is voluntary commitment to
an exercise program known as?

called exercise adherence

TWO: 2 CONCEPT – DEFINITION

cells

organism

microscopic, self-replicating, structural, and functional units of the body that perform many different functions

total collection of all the parts of the biological hierarchy working together to form a living being; largest structure of the biological hierarchy

lateral

bones

osteoporosis

further from the midline of the body

stiff connective tissue found in the human body that protects internal organs, synthesizes blood cells, stores necessary minerals, and provides the muscular system with leverage to produce movement

poor bone mineral density due to low production or loss of adequate calcium content and bone cells, causing bone brittleness

adduction

center of gravity

sliding filament theory

muscular contraction that moves the limbs toward the midline of the body

---

imaginary point on the body at which body weight is completely and evenly distributed in relation to the ground

---

According to this theory, the proteins in muscles, actin, and myosin form a connection to pull the thin actin filaments over the thick myosin filaments. This causes a shortening of the sarcomeres and the concomitant shortening of the muscles, known as muscular contraction.

concentric muscular contraction

delayed onset muscle soreness (DOMS)

mechanical advantage

a muscular contraction when the tension on a muscle is increased as the muscle shortens

a side effect of performing training that overloads the muscles; involves acute muscular soreness caused by micro-tears in the muscle fibers

the efficiency of the lever system based on where the forces are being applied

ATP (Adenosine Triphosphate)

lactate threshold

ball-and-socket joint

the basic energy unit required by the body to perform movement and other metabolic processes

the maximal rate at which lactic acid due to exercise can be buffered from the bloodstream

a joint that allows for range of motion through multiple planes and is comprised of a round bone end and a flat or cup-shaped surface (i.e., the hip and shoulder joints)

supination

macronutrients

lean body mass

joint motion occurring at the forearm during which the palm of the hand is rotated to face upward

---

nutrients that are divided into carbohydrates, proteins, and fats and required by the body in large quantities, typically in the range of tens to hundreds of grams (g) per day

---

part of the body composition calculated by subtracting body fat from body weight; refers to organs, tissues, bones, and muscle (including some fatty tissues, such as the brain and spinal cord)

anabolic steroids

PAR-Q

medical history

These are synthetic compounds that mimic the action of testosterone, the male sex hormone; they stimulate muscular growth and improved athletic performance. Use of anabolic steroids can result in serious side effects, such as irritability, acne, swelling of hands and feet, shrinking of testes in men, growth of facial hair in women, kidney, liver and heart damage.

A physical activity readiness questionnaire (PAR-Q) is used to help personal trainers determine whether individuals have any health, medical, or physical conditions that may prevent them from participating in an exercise program.

This information is collected on a form and pertains to a client's past and present health status, including specific chronic diseases or conditions he or she may suffer from, recent surgeries or injuries, current medications, and more. This information can be helpful in determining if a client requires medical clearance prior to starting an exercise program.

lifestyle questionnaire

relative contraindications

absolute contraindications

This is a form used to determine the activities and habits a client is involved in to determine how to develop the client's training program in a way that suits his or her lifestyle and recreational activities.

These are conditions (i.e., high blood pressure, musculoskeletal injures, history of heart illness, etc.) that affect the client's ability to perform an exercise test, which may be exacerbated by exercise and pose a risk to the client's health.

These are conditions that, due to severity, completely prevent an individual from participating in exercise testing. Such conditions include signs of poor perfusion, dizziness, confusion, light-headedness, sudden onset of chest pain, failure of increased heart rate with an increase in workload, or if the individual requests to stop the testing for any reason.

proprioceptive neuromuscular
facilitation

eccentric muscular contraction

closed kinetic chain

an assisted type of stretching technique that utilizes a static stretch paired with isometric contractions to increase range of motion of a muscle group

a type of muscular contraction during which the muscle resists force while lengthening

exercises in which either the hands or feet remain in contact with a stable surface throughout the range of motion

power

agility

quickness

the ability of the body to move a resistive force rapidly

the ability of the body to rapidly change direction

the ability of the body to react to a cue or stimulus and respond with movement

static stretching

specificity

progression

holding a muscle in a lengthened position for thirty seconds or more to elicit an elongation of the muscle being stretched

developing a training program to achieve a specific goal determined by the trainer and client

an increase in program difficulty through increased frequency and intensity of exercise throughout the client's fitness program

overload

general adaptation syndrome

linear periodization

gradually increasing the difficulty of each successive workout by manipulating the training variables

physiological adaptations to exercise through proper periodization and use of the overload principle

a steady progression toward higher intensity workouts throughout a periodized fitness program

undulating periodization

verbal communication

nonverbal communication

a training program where intensity varies within a microcycle

expression through words

a method of how people express themselves through body language and tone of voice

active listening

visual learner

auditory learner

expressing attentiveness to a conversation through maintaining eye contact, an open body position, and reiterating what the person just said to show understanding

an individual who learns a new skill or information by watching it being performed or through by using other visual aids

an individual who acquires new knowledge by listening to how a skill is performed

kinesthetic learner

external feedback

negligence

an individual who acquires new knowledge by physically performing a skill or activity that represents the information he or she is trying to learn

feedback from outside sources regarding performance evaluation and methods of improvement

failure of a trainer or fitness facility to follow guidelines to properly minimize risks in the training environment

overtraining

FAST

RICE

the body's response to too much physical stress in too short a period of time

---

This is an acronym used for determining if an individual is suffering from a stroke and how to react. The acronym stands for: Face—does one side of the individual's face droop when smiling? Arm—does one arm drift down when the individual tries to raise both arms? Speech— is the individual's speech slurred or strange? Time—if you see any of these signs, dial 911 immediately.

This is an acronym that describes how to administer first aid for musculoskeletal injuries; it stands for: Rest, Ice, Compression, and Elevation.

hyperthermia

hypotension

scope of practice

an abnormally increased body temperature, typically due to exercise in extremely hot and humid climates

an abnormally low blood pressure due to a rapid change in body position or, more seriously, potential heart disease

Scope of practice describes the parameters within which the personal trainer must remain when providing clients with professional information and advice. For instance, personal trainers are within their scope of practice to provide clients with a fitness program; however, it is not within their scope of practice to provide advice regarding medications.

THREE: DEFINITION – CONCEPT

innermost, smooth layer of the heart walls

a muscle that helps create a pressure differential in the abdomen and chest, allowing air to flow into and out of the lungs

endocardium

diaphragm

blood pressure above 140/80 mmHg

two parts of the neuron: the stem-like structures that conduct information to other neurons, and the branching systems on the neuron's body that receive information from other neurons

part of the nervous system associated with the body's ability to control skeletal muscle and voluntary movement as well as involuntary reflexes associated with skeletal muscles

hypertension

axons and dendrites

somatic nervous system

chemical substances that control different bodily and cellular processes; released by glands

a lever system—the most common one in the human body—in which the muscular force is placed closer to the fulcrum than the resistive force

the muscle's ability to apply force to an object, often measured by using a one-repetition maximum test

hormones

third-class lever

strength

an energy source used by the body within the first seconds of exercise to rapidly synthesize ATP

the deleterious effects of over-exercising among female athletes, consisting of three main symptoms: amenorrhea, osteoporosis, and disordered eating habits

contraction of the muscle to move the legs or arms away from the midline of the body

creatine phosphate

the female athlete triad

abduction

joint action at the forearm during which the palm of the hand is turned to face down

excessive posterior curvature of the spine, typically at the thoracic spine

a lever system in which the muscular and resistive forces are on opposite sides of the fulcrum

pronation

kyphosis

first-class lever

the practice of artificially increasing the oxygen-carrying capacity of the blood in order to improve endurance performance (Methods include: blood transfusions, erythropoietin (EPO) injections to stimulate red blood cell production, synthetic oxygen carriers, and cobalt chloride, an illegal method in competitive sports.)

a simple calculation used to determine if individuals are underweight, a healthy weight, overweight, or obese by taking their weight in kilograms (kg) divided by their height in square meters (m^2)

an ergogenic aid used to supplement the PCr (phosphocreatine) levels in the muscle to enhance ATP production in the early stages of an exercise, such as sprinting or weight lifting movements

blood doping

body mass index (BMI)

creatine

the process of determining the importance, size, or value of something through an evaluation or test

the degree to which a test or test item accurately measures information

the consistency or repeatability of a test

assessment

validity

reliability

exercises involving rapid force production in a short period of time (such as jumping, hopping, medicine ball throws, etc.) to develop muscular power

an individual's ability to sense the location of his or her body in space

exercises in a training program involving multiple large muscle groups, such as the quadriceps, hamstrings, glutes, chest, and back musculature

plyometrics

proprioception

core exercises

a breathing technique used to lift heavy loads by forceful exhalation against a sealed airway to create intra-abdominal pressure

utilizing a tool, such as a foam roller, to compress adhesions in the muscle's fascia to promote improvements in range of motion and reduce movement compensations

lying on the stomach

Valsalva maneuver

self-myofascial release (SMR)

prone position

the start of a training program typically associated with lower intensities of exercise with the goal of improving muscular endurance, muscular hypertrophy, and the basic strength of a client

the period during an athlete's event or season defined by peak performance or maintenance of fitness

a goal that is specific, measurable, action-oriented, realistic, and time-stamped

preparatory period

competitive period

SMART goal

a function of the number of sets, repetitions, and exercises in a workout

a calculation involving the client's resting heart rate and estimated maximum heart rate to determine his or her target heart rate zone

the body's deleterious reaction to stopping a training program, evident in as little as two weeks

volume

Karvonen formula

detraining

a decrease in exercise difficulty to accommodate individuals who cannot perform an exercise due to either physical limitations or inexperience

the amount of weight lifted with proper form

the planned breakdown of the overall training program aimed at achieving a specific fitness goal and peak performance; the blueprint of the client's program and how it will be implemented

regression

load

periodization

principle describing the frequency, intensity, time, type, and enjoyment of exercise

the measurement of the body's caloric energy consumption during exercise compared to its consumption at rest

a subjective scale measuring how hard clients feel they are working during exercise

FITTE principle

METs

rate of perceived exertion

utilizing key phrases or specific movements in conjunction with a client's learning style to teach that client how to properly perform an exercise

the ability of an individual to coordinate muscle groups to function cohesively while maintaining spatial awareness

stage of learning during which the client has difficulty performing exercises due to lack of stability, strength, or basic knowledge of the movement pattern

cueing

kinesthetic awareness

cognitive stage

stage of learning during which a client demonstrates a kinesthetic connection to the exercise and is able to stabilize his or her body to perform the exercise with minimal compensation

stage of learning during which the client has a clear understanding of how the exercise is performed and requires a progression of the same exercise to present a challenge

internal motivating factors for self-improvement (i.e., starting a fitness program for general health benefits)

associative stage

autonomous stage

intrinsic motivation

external motivating factors for self-improvement (i.e., a class reunion or beach season)

an increased breathing rate that occurs at rest and is potentially a sign of a cardiac or pulmonary emergency

a form used to outline the details of the exercise testing procedures and training program to affirm the client was informed of these prior to participation in exercise

extrinsic motivation

hyperventilation

informed consent form

low blood sugar, potentially leading to slurred speech, dizziness, confusion, sweating, loss of coordination, fatigue, irritability, tachycardia, blurred vision, and syncope

fainting due to metabolic conditions

term referring to a network of licensed, certified, or registered professionals who provide invaluable healthcare resources to the general population

hypoglycemia

syncope

allied healthcare continuum

9 781635 303698